Taking Back Control

How to Keep a Firm Grip on Your Emotions, and Achieve Balance in Your Life

Nicky Curtis

Contents

Introduction

"It's just emotions taking me over ..." once sang Destiny's Child (or the Bee Gees, depending on which era you were born in), in a song closely related to heartbreak and pining over a former lover. You're singing along to it in your head right now, aren't you?

Well, whether you relate it to the actual song's meaning, or you take the words for what they are, there is a very real case to state that emotions can indeed take you over in their entirety, if you let them.

Welcome to the world of emotions – sometimes difficult, sometimes joyous, and sometimes there is no adjective to actually describe them. If you are constantly feeling like you are battling the way you feel, then this book is for you.

Have you ever felt so completely drowned in the way you were feeling? Have you ever felt like you have a brick resting in the bottom of your stomach, feeling sick all the time? Do you want to cry for no apparent reason, or do you feel like you're simply down and can't drag yourself back up?

These are all very common, and very legitimate, feelings that are linked to emotional issues in our lives.

Everyone has emotions, whether you believe it or not - yes, that person who appears heartless, he or she still feels things, but perhaps he or she is just better at hiding them than you are. Put simply, emotions are an intrinsic part of human nature; we feel because we are human, we feel because we care, we feel because we are supposed to, what we are not supposed to do however is let these emotions dictate our lives to a negative, because that is a spiralling road towards depression, anxiety, and a huge hindrance to success on many levels. If you want a successful life, you have to put in the time and effort to conquer those sometimes difficult situations – but, you can do it!

Some of us are simply more emotional than others, but that isn't a failing, not if you can control those emotions and harness them for good, to fulfil the potential in your life. Whilst nobody ever said it was easy, and it really isn't, with practice, turning a negative into a positive, and a difficult situation into something to be proud of, this can all become much easier, and much more do-able on a regular basis. Nobody ever goes through life without encountering problems or hard times, but the key is to focus on the good, rather than the bad.

This book is for people just like you – people who perhaps struggle to keep an even keel on the way they are feeling, people who find that their emotions are easily thrown out of sync whenever a troubling situation arises. Our emotions play such a huge part in our lives, that if we don't get the balance right, it can affect our happiness and success in both work and relationships, to name just two areas. Life is a balance, and when one part of our life is out of sync, it basically throws the rest of it off kilter too – achieve a balance and you will feel much more grounded, and indeed much more content as a result.

Because of all of this, it is important to assess our emotional make up, to find out the degree to which we feel things, and to see how this affects our general health and wellbeing. When you have this answer, you are in a much better position to make sure that you don't let your emotions dictate your life, or even rule your life, in a negative way.

If you're reading this and wondering what all this mumbo jumbo is about, well, that mumbo jumbo really does mean something! Emotions are powerful things, and to the degree where they can occasionally render a person useless – don't let that be you!

In this book we will show you the tools to help you effectively manage your emotions, giving you strategies and information on how to channel your feelings for the good in your life, without letting them pull you down towards the dark, swirling mess that is negativity. Nobody needs negativity in their life! Think about that person at work who always seems to be frowning, does anyone really want to be around them? Not really! Now think about the person who is always smiling, are they popular? Yes! Be that happy and popular person, not the one who could give Eeyore a run for their money.

If you're reading this and nodding your head, thinking "yes! That's me!" well, good news is about to come your way; if you're reading this and thinking "what the hell is all this about?" well, read on to find out! Emotions are a mystery, that's for sure, but they are certainly interesting, and certainly can be harnessed if you know how to go about it.

Chapter 1: Taking a Look Inwards: What Are Emotions?

Okay, so you've picked up this book because of several different reasons, these could be:

- You are interested in the differences between emotions and feelings
- You feel a lot, and you are keen to figure out how to handle it all for a positive
- You are eager to learn how to read other people's emotions, to develop your own interpersonal skills
- Emotions interest you
- Any of the above

Put simply, emotions are one of the key reasons we are human, because every single human being on the planet feels certain things, be it love, hate, or greed, trust, panic, joy, or fear. These are just several examples of certain types of emotion you may feel at any time during your life. It's important to realise that there is a difference between an emotion and a mood:

An emotion is a feeling, a reaction to a situation or experience in your life, which is generally short-lived.

A mood is more of a general feeling which lasts for a much longer period of time, such as frustration, unhappiness, happiness, sadness, or anxiety.

Once you figure this difference out, you're on a much better level to understand what emotions are. Whilst emotions certainly aren't an exact science, there is some measuring to be done in a laboratory, to a degree.

Scientists have had a hard time figuring out emotions, because let's face it, how do you really measure an emotion? One person's idea of how love feels could be totally different to how the other person in the relationship feels, but that doesn't mean they love the person any less, they simply interpret the feeling and emotion differently. It's complicated, as you can see! Every single person in the world is an individual, and that means that everyone feels things in a slightly different, subtle way.

This is probably what makes emotions so interesting, but also so complex. If you really look at feelings and emotions from a distance, they are intriguing, to say the least, but when you are feeling them to a strong degree, you could probably be forgiven for wondering where the 'off' switch is – well, the bad news is that there isn't such a switch, but there is a way to turn them down a little.

Every single person on the planet has emotions, but how to study them or even how to measure them, is a difficult one to go with. There are however three different parts to any single emotion, be it love, guilt, jealousy, upset, fear, confusion, or hate, for example:

- Subjective emotions or feelings
- Physical responses to emotions or feelings
- Expressive components to emotions or feelings

Let's look at each one in turn, to help you understand how your mind and body react to each emotion you feel.

Subjective emotions or feelings

We mentioned in our last section about everyone having a different idea about how something feels, such as two people who are going through a grief process – one person may deal with it better than the other, but it doesn't mean they're not hurting as much. One person may find it easier to talk about how they feel, to express their emotions more outwardly, but the other person may find themselves paralysed in terms of vocalising it all; this is a subjective reaction to an emotion or feeling. The same can be said for two people in a relationship – one person might love the hearts and flowers side of things, feeling that this is what love is all about; the other person might simply feel that spending time together is enough, and these differences in perspective are what make up our subjective reactions to that feeling.

You can't measure a subjective emotion or feeling reaction because it's about talking about how you feel, and as we just mentioned, everyone describes the feeling differently. This is the part of measuring emotions that scientists basically hate, because there is no way to figure it out!

Physical responses to emotions or feelings

Okay, this is the side of things which is much easier to figure out for those wanting to measure emotions. This is the way your body reacts to the way you are feeling; for example, when you are feeling embarrassed about something, you blush, and this is blood rushing to the surface of the skin on your face – this is a physical reaction to an emotion. Other common reactions include:

- A racing heart
- Shaking
- Sweating
- An additional feeling of panic

- An adrenaline release
- Tearfulness
- Being unable to get your words out
- Clumsiness
- Feeling completely distracted in the moment

This is all tied into the old caveman 'fight or flight' response, which was basically developed in order to keep us safe when faced with a situation that deep down we fear is harmful. This is all about the release of the adrenaline hormone, and this is what causes that thumping heart and shaking feeling; don't worry, it's all perfectly normal, and it's your body's way of keeping you safe in the face of what it perceives to be a dangerous or hurtful situation.

Expressive components to emotions or feelings

Again, scientists love this side of things, because there is a measure to be had, and this allows them to study that confusing mess we call emotions!

Put simply, even if you are an Oscar-worthy actor or actress, there is no way of hiding from a physical or expressive reaction to an emotion or feeling. A little like a physical reaction, an expressive reaction is all about body language, which we display sometimes without even realising it.

You've probably heard a lot about body language in terms of expressing yourself in a certain way, e.g. in a job interview, for example, but when it comes to a reaction to an emotion, we act a certain way without even realising it, sometimes paralysed by the emotion we are feeling. For instance, if you hear something hurtful, your face is likely to drop without you even knowing it, and that gives the other person in the situation a clue that they have said something to you which has affected the way you feel.

Other expressive reactions include:

- Raised eyebrows
- A pause for breath
- Shocked breath
- Crying (either happy or sad tears)
- Freezing
- Tense muscles
- A change in the voice tone
- Closed body language, e.g. arms crossed over the body

If you can learn to recognise these reactive behaviors then this will really help you develop your interpersonal skills, when dealing with other people. Basically, you're looking for clues on how someone is feeling.

Why do we have emotions?

We've mentioned that we feel emotions because we are basically human, but why?

Talk about a difficult question to answer!

We feel because we are meant to, this is something which scientists generally agree on; the way we feel emotions is a big part of what makes us different from one another – if we were all the same, life would be extremely boring, after all.

It's for this reason that you need to learn to embrace your emotions, rather than be at war with them, and this book will help you do just that.

Think about it – have you ever heard a particular song on the radio and immediately been transported back to a time in your head, something you experienced before? The emotions you felt at that time will probably be felt too, albeit a little less harshly than at the time it happened. Smells and certain tastes are powerful reminders of times gone by too. These are potential triggers for an emotion, however more likely a memory.

All this is explained basically by that flight or fight reaction we talked about briefly earlier in this chapter. Emotions are there to keep you alive, to save you from troublesome situations, and to help you realise that there is a potential danger at hand. For example, just to make this a little easier to understand, if you feel fear then this is your body's way of trying to keep you safe, which explains why we tend to freeze in scary situations.

Whilst this doesn't answer the question of why we have emotions that comprehensively, this is the line which scientists are generally going down. Put simply, not all emotions can be explained that way, because falling in love is an emotion, and the explanation doesn't really fit this mould. Probably one of the best ways to explain why we feel things in this way is with this four word sentence – we just don't know!

Maybe that's what is so wonderful about the vast array of emotions we feel as human beings, both good and bad, because this is what sets us apart, what makes us different, and basically, what makes life worth living. Can you imagine a life without emotions? Can you imagine not feeling anything?

Whether you're plagued by negative emotions in your life, thinking about it this way really does put it into perspective – feeling something is always better than feeling nothing, and is much better than total numbness, provided you can learn how to manage your negative emotions and turn them into something much more positive.

There's an awful lot of debate about this, and much of it comes down to whether you are a sensitive person or not. You could also put some of this down to horoscopes, if you believe that kind of thing.

Cancerians are said to be extremely sensitive souls, and are also believed to be ruled by the moon, which is responsible for turbulent and sometimes extreme emotions.

Do you believe this?

Whether you do or not, there are many people who give some credit to this claim.

Basically, it's best to say it this way – everyone feels to some degree or another, but perhaps those who claim to not feel as much have simply learnt to manage and balance their emotions better than those who feel consumed by them, regardless of their star sign.

This chapter is designed to give you a brief overview of what an emotion is, because once you understand what it is we are talking about, and you understand that an emotion is very different to a mood, you can begin to identify your particular emotional problems, and put into place ways to manage them. Throughout this book we will give you the tools and strategies to do just that, and with the brief knowledge we have discussed in this chapter, you are now ready to progress onto step number two.

Chapter 2: Check Your Emotions – Your Personal Emotional Check List

Everyone has a degree to which emotions rule their lives, whether it is to a small degree, because they have an emotional capacity to keep everything in check, or whether it is to a large degree, because they are a very sensitive person, who can easily allow their emotions to dictate their life. Of course, there are people who are in-between, the ones who have achieved balance – this is your aim!

Throughout this book we are giving you advice, tips, and information on how to control and maintain your emotions on an even keel, without letting an extreme on one side come into play. Balance is your aim, and balance is what you shall have!

Okay, first things first, before we get onto strategies and handy tips on how to achieve balance, we need to get a heads up on how much you 'feel'. The check list below will help you identify your personal emotional capacity, with a few scenarios to put you in situations which may spike emotions or feelings.

See how you fare with the scenarios below, and check your results against the explanations.

Scenario 1
You are in a relationship, a quite serious relationship, and you feel that your partner is being distant. You're not sure why this is happening, but you don't like it, that's for sure. What is your line of thinking?

1) You immediately think you have done something wrong, scanning your brain for your actions over the last few days, and trying to identify what the issue could

be. You become tearful and blame yourself for your partner's mood.

2) You shrug it off and put it down to a situation which you don't know about. You haven't done anything wrong, that's all you know.

3) You ask your partner if there is anything wrong, and offer to listen. You know there is nothing on your side that is wrong, and you know that when they are ready to discuss their worries, they will come to you. In the meantime you simply try and do nice things for them.

Analysis

If you chose option 1 then you are a highly emotional and highly sensitive person. If you chose option 3, you are balanced – well done! If you chose option 2 then you are possibly a little too on the side of uncaring; not necessarily a bad thing to be aware that you haven't done anything wrong, but consideration on the other person's side is a must have.

In this situation, if you know you haven't done anything to cause the problem, and you have asked what is wrong and received a non-response, then really you should let this drop and allow your thoughts to be calm. The person will come to your side when they ready to talk, so simply be patient.

Scenario 2

A colleague at work has taken credit for a project which you largely contributed to. Quite rightly, you feel hard done by, and you feel angry, but how extreme is your reaction? Be honest about how you would react to this scenario, and put aside the way you think you would react in your head – stick to reality.

1) You keep everything inside whilst at work, but silently rage and seethe when you are at home, with your loved

ones. You feel extremely betrayed and that this situation is unfair and unjust.

2) You lose your temper at work, telling the person exactly how you feel about it, and speaking to your boss about the situation. Why shouldn't you get the credit for the work you did?

3) You approach the person concerned and try in the calmest way possible to ask why they did this. You are obviously upset, and you are feeling anything but calm, but you attempt to keep an even keel and get the explanation.

Analysis

This is a difficult situation to manage emotions-wise, because you are completely right in feeling ridiculed and that the outcome is totally unfair. Of course, you did the work too, so you should also receive some of the praise. The key in this situation however is to remain calm, and not to allow your emotions to get the better of you. Anger is a feeling, an emotion, and when you feel hard done by, it's very easy to let that overcome all sense and reason, potentially putting you in a more difficult situation than you were in before.

If you chose option number 1 then you have pretty much allowed yourself to be walked all over, and this is a sign of holding your emotions inside too much. If you choose option number 2, again this an extreme reaction in the opposite direction. Going in all guns blazing is not a good way to manage the situation, and that means you allowed your anger and feeling of justice not being served to take over your mind and sense of reason for a short time.

So, that leaves us with option number 3; this is the option which displays balanced emotions. Of course, you are feeling unhappy about it, you are angry, and you know the situation is wrong, but you have managed to see calm in the storm, and you have approached it in the same way – this is the option which is most likely to get you the best outcome in the end.

Scenario 3

You are having a bad day; everything seems to be going wrong, everything you try and fix backfires, and nobody seems to understand your predicament. Put simply, you wish you had stayed in bed. To what degree do you allow your emotions to affect your day?

1) You try and laugh at everything that goes wrong, even though it is hard to do. You appreciate that things go wrong sometimes, but you can't help but wonder if you got out of bed the wrong side that morning.
2) You break down in tears after the first few mishaps and wonder what you did to the world to deserve such a bad day.
3) You feel angry and want to throw everything on the floor and scream. Anyone who comes near you is likely to get a tongue-lashing, and you simply don't want to engage in conversation with anyone.

Analysis

Everyone has bad days, this is just a simple fact of life; the trick is to not allow it to completely ruin your day and to turn everyone against you in the process. Your reaction to this simple 'one of those things' situations will give you a lot of information on how much you allow your reactions to dictate your life.

If you chose option number 1, well done, you're trying your best not to get stressed, but this could also display a rather 'whatever' kind of attitude. You need to at least care a little! Option number 2 is the one you will have chosen if you are a sensitive soul, someone who is upset easily. Yes, your day isn't desirable, but unfortunately it has happened, and crying for long over spilt milk is not going to help matters. Option number 3 displays behaviour of those who turn their problems into aggression, and this displays emotional overreactions opposite to those displayed by sensitive people.

The key here, the way to achieve balance, is to sit somewhere in the middle of all of these three options – don't allow yourself to become complacent, yes, laugh, it's something that happens, don't cry about it for longer than a couple of minutes (it's not the end of the world, after all), and don't turn your emotional stress into aggression and anger.

These are just three scenarios, but you can see quite clearly from the answers to choose from the way in which this explanation is going.

You are basically either:

a) Too emotional
b) Not emotional enough
c) Balanced

Of course, there are people who are in the middle of all that, and this either means you are approaching balance, or you are too far in the opposite direction. The answers you gave to these three simple scenarios should have identified your particular emotional type.

If you are type A, e.g. over-emotional, then this means you will have answered the scenarios in a way that showed you take everything to heart, you think everything is your fault, and you cry or become upset very easily.

Now, don't worry if this is you, because there is nothing wrong with being sensitive, it's actually a gift to be so in tune with your emotions and the way you can easily understand others, but if you allow it to dictate your life, you could find yourself spiralling into the dark and murky waters of depression and anxiety. Remember that the world is not out to get you, and that your emotions can easily be kept in check if you continue reading this book, and learn the tricks of the trade.

If you are type B, e.g. loosely described as not being emotional enough, don't worry either! We are not for a second suggesting that you lack emotional intelligence, or that you lack feeling; you are certainly not heartless, you are simply less likely to outwardly show what you are feeling to others, and instead you allow your emotions to get the better of you in a more negative way, e.g. emotional outbursts in the form of anger and shouting.

The key here is to think calm thoughts! If you explode every single time something gets to you, people are simply not going to want to be around you, it's that simple. Keep the situation in perspective, and think before you react.

Finally, we have type C, the balanced types. This is, as we have mentioned, the type you are aiming to be. Balanced types are emotional, but they are also under-emotional at the same time; they simply know when to show what they are feeling, how to do it, and the degree to which it happens. Some people are born this way, others learn to be this way, but basically, being balanced means your life will be in harmony, and you are less likely to suffer because of emotional outbursts or upsets.

Now you understand the degree to which you react in situations, you know which way you need to work, and you can work towards that goal with the helpful advice we're going to talk about.

Chapter 3: An Impossible Explanation? Figuring out Your Emotions

We know what emotions are now, we know that they are feelings which are associated with a certain event or situation, basically something which has happened, and we know that they are usually quite short lived. If the feeling goes on for longer, this is usually referred to as a mood, which is a reactive state of mind.

Okay, so we know what an emotion is, and whilst we talked about the fact that scientists love to try and put them in a box and explain them in a logical way, this is not always entirely possible. Emotions are human things, they are a state of feeling which we have because we are flesh and blood, and whilst they can be painful and upsetting sometimes, they can also be wonderful things too – it's like the old 'what goes up, must come down' theory, everything good in life is balanced out with something not so good.

Knowing what an emotion is forms only a small part of the story however, because in order to be able to figure out why you feel the way you do, and therefore manage and control your emotions to create a positive in your life, we need to understand what affects emotions, and what causes you as an individual to feel a certain way.

What affects emotions?

We will talk about emotional triggers in a lot more detail in a later chapter, because everyone's triggers are different, however for now, we'll explore what can actually affect an emotion, e.g. what can affect the way you feel.

Think about your daily routine for example, do you feel statically the same throughout the day? It's unlikely, and if you do, well, you could actually be a robot! No, you are more likely to experience a range of emotions throughout a 24 hours' period, and whilst some people will feel them more intensely than others, everyone feels them to some degree.

Understanding your emotions can be as complicated as the Matrix, however figuring out how you feel, such as taking the time out to ask yourself 'how do I feel about this', is a good stepping stone.

So, what can affect your emotions?

- A situation which makes you feel uncomfortable, something which hurts you, something which you are not sure of, or something you are unhappy about.
- Another person – for instance, a person who we may refer to as a 'mood hooverer'. Yes, we mentioned moods are different to emotions, but have you ever experienced that one person who simply sucks the entire life out of you when you walk into the room? We will refer to that rather sour-faced person as a 'mood hooverer', or perhaps an 'energy vampire'; whatever you call them, you get the jist.
- Fear of a situation which has not yet happened, or possibly won't ever happen. Come on, you've surely experienced a 'what if' kind of deal, and these are sometimes the worst things for making anxiety spike. The key with this situation is to realise that it hasn't happened yet, and maybe it never will. In the short-term however, this can be a worrying emotion to experience.
- A work problem, something which causes you more of an irritation than an actual anger.

- Falling in love or being in a relationship. There can be both positive and negative emotions attached to love, and of course we want it to be hearts and flowers, but life simply isn't a Disney movie all the time. You can feel on top of the world when you're in love, and this is an emotion, or you can feel mixed up and unsure, and again, that is an emotion too.
- A job interview or situation where you need to prove yourself. This can cause nerves, which are a very valid emotion. Dealing with nerves is the same thing as learning to control emotions, because nerves can be as debilitating as a negative emotion.
- A string of positive events. Emotions aren't negatives all the time! Whilst we are probably going to talk about how to deal with negative emotions mostly throughout this book, because they are the ones which can cause the most distress, it's important to point out that there is a flip side of the coin too – positive emotions, such as happiness, feeling on top of the world, and feeling lucky or content, perhaps even excited for the future, these are all emotions which can be caused by happy events in your life.
- A situation in which you aren't 100% sure of the facts. Confusion and not knowing where you stand can spike your emotions, and this can cause you to stop eating, feel nervous, lose sleep etc.

The list of what can affect emotions goes on, because we are all individuals, and what causes one person to feel happiness, might cause another person to feel simply okay; what causes one person to want to cry, might cause one person to simply shrug it all off.

Again, this can be personal, but on the whole there are certain situations which bring up similar feelings and emotions within all of us. For instance, if you are cheated on in a relationship, you will no doubt feel hurt, anger, confusion, as the main emotions coming to the fore; if you are about to go to a job interview you will probably be feeling fear, anxiety, maybe confusion too.

As you can see, certain situations are common emotional triggers, which we will discuss in much more detail in an upcoming chapter. The main point of this section however is to get you to see that if you feel a certain way about a certain situation, you shouldn't think that what you are feeling is wrong in any way, your emotions are yours, but what you shouldn't do is let them own you.

The tools to really deal with emotions are about to be revealed, however it's important for us to say now that these first few chapters are about getting you to understand why we feel emotions, and what they are in the first place. If you don't have a clue what something is, how can you understand it? It's like swimming through mud – basically impossible!

The point to take from this chapter, if you didn't get anything else (and if not, why not?) is that emotions are there for a reason, because you are human and because the situation you are going through evokes a human response.

In the words of Human League, 'I'm only human, of flesh and blood I'm made ...'

If that's before your time, ask your mum!

Chapter 4: Danger, danger! What Happens When You Allow Emotions to Dictate Your Life

Most of us like to think of ourselves as independent sorts, nobody really likes to admit that they rely on other people to get by in life. Do you agree with that? Most of you should probably be nodding your heads right now.

Basically, whilst we like to think we're all singing, all dancing, fiercely independent types, the truth of the matter is that most of us flounder from time to time, be it because of a problematic situation in our lives, relationships, work etc, or because of a situation that we just don't really know how to deal with.

Put simply, it's okay to struggle from time to time, it's okay to let your emotions out, in fact, believe it or not, letting your emotions out is actually healthy! Without wanting to sound overly Oprah about all of this, if you allow yourself to become blocked, if you bottle everything up and turn into a ticking time bomb, then really all that's ever going to happen is an explosion of some sort.

The late, great Oscar Wilde once put all of this into perfect perspective with one quote - "I don't want to be at the mercy of my emotions. I want to use them, to enjoy them, and to dominate them".

Who could word it better?

Your emotions are there for a reason, as we have mentioned time and time again; you are human, you feel, this is normal, however what is not normal is to allow those feelings to dictate your life. There are very real dangers to allowing that to happen.

Let this be a set of bullet pointed warnings:

- Depression
- Anxiety
- Becoming that aforementioned 'mood hooverer' yourself
- Feeling desperate, like there is no future to look forward to
- Lack of appetite, loss of weight
- Affected health
- Alienating yourself from your loved ones
- Damaging relationships
- Problems at work
- Distractions/an inability to focus
- Lack of hope
- Complete and utter negativity

These are just a few of the problems which being a slave to your emotions can cause; it's best to stop at this point, without wanting to depress you entirely. As you can see, there is nothing good to come out of being ruled by a feeling or emotion, and instead there is everything good about taking the other option – learning to control it all.

Being emotional isn't always a bad thing …

Don't fall into the trap of thinking that being an emotional person is a negative thing, a bad thing even, because that's not the truth. Being an emotional person is a positive too, because you can learn to become more self-aware, you open yourself up to experiences and feelings, you can develop empathy, and help others too, and you are likely to be a very good listener as a result. On the flip side however, being too emotional means you are likely to find melancholy in everything.

An out of balance set of emotions for a long period of time can lead to depression, anxiety, poor health, problems in relationships and work, and a constant stream of negativity in terms of your thoughts can also simply be a downward spiral that is not fun at all. There is no 'scream if you want to go faster' about this ride, it's basically 'let me off!'

Of course, you can be emotional in stages, i.e. you are normally quite reserved, but a certain situation in your life causes you to be more emotional than you normally would be. This is entirely normal, and is called being emotional reactively. Even the hardest person on the planet can get upset and worried from time to time, perhaps because of an issue with their job, in their relationship, or because of the loss of a loved one. Whilst these strong emotions might be short-lived, they are certainly intense at the time, especially if that person isn't used to being quite so emotional all the time.

Someone who is overly emotional all of the time however can become tired of it all. Imagine the scene – you are constantly feeling every emotion under the sun throughout the day, and you feel like everything is going wrong. When you feel negative emotions, they can be draining, especially if it is a case of up and down all the time. That person then simply wants to sleep a lot, because it means they shut it all out and they don't feel as much – perfectly reasonable, but definitely not healthy.

If this sounds like a scenario you're quite familiar with, you are certainly more towards the emotional end of the scale.

Okay, so we've talked about what happens when you allow emotions to take over your entire being, and we've mentioned how it can affect you negatively; we have also said that emotions aren't a bad thing, and that it's important to find balance in your life, to enable you to use your emotions to spur you on to greater things, perhaps success in a job, or going for it with that person you have loved secretly for years. Now we will go on to talk about what can trigger severe emotional responses, before talking about how you can use those emotions for a positive, and how you can harness their power and stop them from negatively affecting your life, or even simply your day!

Chapter 5: Pulling The Trigger – Common Emotional Hot Spots

Your emotions don't spike for no particular reason, and if they do, well, you need to look at exactly why your emotions are that unpredictable. On the whole however, an emotion or feeling is triggered because of a situation, circumstance, or a separate feeling within you. Figuring out what that trigger is means you can start to control the situation, but when you are in the heat of the moment, that can be difficult.

Think about it, when you are upset about something, perhaps you have seen your boyfriend or girlfriend getting a little too cosy with someone else, are you likely to be able to chill out and think before reacting? Unlikely!

If you are that controlled then, seriously, well done, but on the whole, most of us would react first and think later. If you do fall into that latter category, don't beat yourself up about it, because you are in the majority here. Of course, we have picked a rather extreme situation there, but it is a good example of how you can easily allow your reactions to an emotional trigger to take hold very quickly.

Your personal emotional triggers are something you need to think about, because perhaps there is one thing in your life which kick-starts your emotions more than anything else; it could be something small like being ignored in a queue on the bus, or it could be something big, like the example we just talked about. Once you know your triggers, you can work on minimising the effects.

As a human being, we basically react to how we feel, so if we see something, we feel something, and we react. If you can catch yourself before you react, or at least before you reactions go too far, then you can assess whether or not the trigger is actually real, or whether you are about to throw a huge overreaction. Let's face it, overreactions are a bit on the embarrassing side; we've all done it in the past, and we've all felt a little foolish afterwards!

It all really comes down to that fight or flight theory we were talking about right at the start of the book. When our caveman and woman ancestors were running away from all manner of scary beasts, they trusted their instincts and emotions to dictate what they did. If they felt fear, they reacted by running or fighting, and that is basically what we still do today. You can be grateful that we didn't hold onto some of our former ancestors' other traits, and instead kept this one, which keeps us alive!

It's important to realise that an emotional trigger is not the emotion itself, it is the action, situation, or circumstance, even a feeling, which triggers our emotions and causes our reaction, whatever that may be.

On the whole, some of the main emotional triggers which are common in most of us include:

- Feeling ignored
- Feeling belittled
- Not being accepted
- Being over-looked
- Not being understood
- Feeling out of control in a situation
- Money problems
- Work issues
- Relationship problems

- A lack of attention in a situation, perhaps at work or in your relationship
- Disrespect
- Not being right (we are human after all!)
- Feeling uncomfortable for some reason
- Annoyance or anger at an inability to do something, e.g. a shy person may become angry at themselves because they find it hard to socialise as freely as someone who is more of an extrovert
- Feeling unbalanced
- Being disliked and not understanding why
- Not feeling valued
- Not being treated fairly
- A lack of justice being served in a situation, be it for yourself or someone else
- Feeling trapped, as though you don't have freedom in a situation
- Feeling stuck, e.g. you may feel that life has become predictable, or you are stuck in a rut
- Anything to do with love (yes, it's great, but it also hurts!)
- Dealing with a person who you simply don't like
- Fear of anything
- Worry about a situation, be it worrying for a reason or not – overthinking is a prime reason for emotional triggers

If you read that list and began nodding your head – good news, you're perfectly normal! Most people can relate to most of the situations or feelings on that list, and most people would agree that they are common triggers on a personal level.

What to do when you encounter a trigger

You might read this following section and think 'yeah, yeah, easier said than done', and at first, yes that is true; what you need to remember however is that everything gets easier with practice, and once you can identify your triggers and begin to calm yourself, before you react and raise merry hell, then you will be in a much better position to begin controlling those emotions.

Yes, it sounds confusing, yes it sounds borderline impossible, but yes, it can be done!

Step 1: Think about your triggers

Is there something in your life which annoys you? Something which hurts you? Something which makes you feel fearful, or even angry? This is a trigger for you, because if it stirs up emotions every single time you encounter it, then that is a personal trigger which you need to begin to work on.

For this step, you need to sit down with a pen and paper, and be completely and utterly honest. You also need a clear mind, so put down that glass of wine! Think carefully, run through your day in your mind, did something bother you? Did your emotions come into play and cause a reaction? Write down exactly what caused you to feel that way.

Now you have identified one or two triggers, cast your mind a little further, perhaps over your last few days, or your last week, and then think even further about any recurring situations in your life which cause you to feel a certain way. Write these down.

At the end of this exercise you should have a list of several triggers, your personal emotional trigger points. Now to work on them.

Step 2: Why does this particular trigger cause your emotions to come to the fore?

Again, this is going to take some thinking about. Is it a certain person who triggers your feelings and emotions? Is it work? Is it your relationship? Give some thought into why you allow this situation to affect you to the degree it does. Is there anything you can do to stop this reaction, or is there anything you can do to minimise the effects all, then work on it over time?

If you can identify why something bothers you, then you can start to do something about its impact, and minimise your reactions.

Step 3: Why do you react the way you do?

Okay the next step after figuring out why your trigger affects you, is to figure out why you react the way you do. Do you get angry and throw things? Do you shout at someone? Do you cry? Do you go into yourself and allow worry and overthinking to take over? Pinpoint what your reaction is, and then be realistic about how extreme your reaction is too. Once you have this information you can move onto step number 4.

Step 4: Put some mindful thinking into action

Now you have your list of triggers, you have thought about the degree to which you are affected, the degree to which you react, and you know why you allow the trigger to affect you, it's time to try and do something about it!

When you encounter your particular trigger, or triggers, be aware of it, make sure you are present in the moment and you recognise that you are actually encountering the problem that causes your emotions to spike. You can even say it to yourself if it helps, say something like 'this is my trigger' (although obviously avoid saying it out loud unless you don't mind some strange looks from people!), and this will help you be in the moment, and keep your emotions at bay for at least a few seconds longer.

Now your trigger has been recognised, take a deep breath; breathe in through your nose, hold it for a few seconds, and then breathe out through your mouth – slowly! Repeat it again if you need to. This should help you process what is happening, delaying your reaction, if it actually happens at all. Detach yourself from the trigger, and try and see the situation for what it is – do you really need to get yourself into a state over it? Is there an alternative course of action?

You may notice that you start to display physical signs here, so be aware of those too, and if you sense your muscles tensing, try and relax, close your eyes for a second, and feel the tension leaving your body.

Finally, keep a perspective. You may find that delaying your reaction to your trigger by following these few simple steps can help you assess it and avoid the usual emotional reaction that follows. If you do react anyway, don't worry too much, this is something which takes practice, and there could be a few false starts before you really get to grips with it properly.

Step 5: Assess the situation after the storm has passed
Give it a few minutes, or possibly a few hours, before you sit down and think about how you did. Did you manage to resist your emotions being too much to deal with? Did you manage to avoid your trigger at all? Did you manage to avoid the reaction?

Don't beat yourself up about having this trigger, and don't be upset if you didn't manage to control your emotions this particular time. It's perfectly normal and acceptable to have something in your life which makes you feel uncomfortable or emotional in some way, what matters is that you are aware of it and you try and do something about it if it is affecting you too negatively.

This is the first of our scenarios and exercises which help give you some practical advice in order to get a handle on your emotions, and achieve the balance we are all craving. In the coming chapters we will run through more practical scenarios, and hopefully by the end of this book, you will be a practised master in the art of avoiding awkward, upsetting, or embarrassing situations, which cause your emotions to fly through the roof, and your reaction to follow suit.

Chapter 6: Outbursts and melt-downs, how to deal with a serious emotional tantrum

Sometimes we just explode; yes, it's embarrassing afterwards, yes, you might want the ground to open up and swallow you, and yes, it's potentially distressing if you actually end up saying something you regret to someone you care about, but the bottom line is that our emotions are easily piqued if we are feeling out of sorts, and in that case, an outburst, melt-down, or even tantrum can occur.

Don't worry if this happens - this is life! The thing you need to do however is to think about how often you have these meltdowns, and try and pinpoint the reason why. Is it about one particular situation in your life? If so, you need to get to work on resolving that, or at least minimising its effects. If it's something different every time, are you feeling generally stressed out? Do you find that your anger or emotions bubble very easily? Again, there is likely to be a situation in your life, or a trigger, which is causing an underlying problem, and the first step to sorting it out is to identify what it is.

Of course, you might also be finding that you're in the middle of an emotional melt-down from a loved one or friend, and you might not know how to deal with it.

This chapter will explore what causes a melt-down, why we have them, what we can do about them whilst we're having them, and what to do if someone else is having one. As with our previous chapters, it's really about identifying the trigger, but when you're in the heat of the moment, and your emotions are bubbling like a volcano about to erupt, thinking clearly can be a tad bit difficult!

Don't beat yourself up about it if you find these melt-downs happening occasionally, instead, think about why, and put the following steps and advice into practice.

Why do we have emotional melt-downs?

When we talk about emotional melt-downs, we're not just talking about a slight stress, or feeling an emotion for a few minutes, we're talking about the point that an emotion becomes too much, and it takes over and grabs hold of your general being for a short while. This generally happens because of something which is bothering you, and you might not even be aware of it at the time; your sub-conscious can be a very powerful thing!

The actual reason why you're having this melt-down is personal, because as is the case with anything emotion-related, it's about you as an individual, and what is affecting you at the time. If you are stressed about work, and something else in your life annoys you slightly, you might find that you simply explode, because that underlying work issue is in the back of your mind, waiting to suddenly come to the fore. It's a little like referred pain, e.g. if you have a pain in your back, you might feel it in your shoulder as a referred type of pain, and in the case of emotions, you have a work issue, but you might feel in the form of someone bumping into you in the street by accident, which simply sparks off a chain of emotional reactions – e.g. shouting, stamping the floor etc.

Of course, none of this is healthy, because you're not dealing with the problem at hand, and running away from issues never did anyone any good. What an emotional melt-down really is, is a warning sign – this is your mind or body's way of saying 'this is getting too much, please deal with it', so it's your duty to listen.

If you find yourself in the midst of an emotional drama, where your general emotional feelings come to the fore and are difficult to deal with, you will probably find it hard to really think straight in the moment. The key here is to recognise that you are actually experiencing a melt-down, because then you can rationalise what you are thinking.

Close your eyes for a second or two
Being in the moment is the only real way to understand that you are about to react in a way that might not be the best possible solution to the issue. Think about it – if you shout at someone, you might say something you don't mean, and that is going to take some sorting out. Trying to avoid the reaction in the first place, or at least cut it down, is the key to avoiding a melt-down. So, close your eyes and breathe for a few seconds; this will give you time to calm a little, and hopefully avoid the problem.

Try and identify the emotion you are feeling
Is it anger? Is it upset? Is it disappointment? Try and identify the emotion which is coming to the fore and threatening to bubble out of control. Once you know what it is you're feeling, can you identify why you are feeling it?

Walk away, walk away!
Nobody is suggesting you run away from the problem, but walking away and giving yourself time to calm is the best solution in the short-term. Most of the time, an emotional melt-down is short-lived, and afterwards you might feel a little foolish or embarrassed at the way you allowed your emotions to take hold and dictate your reactions to the extreme that a melt-down allows. If you can give yourself a little time to

assess the situation, you are more likely to see sense, therefore avoiding the melt-down from actually happening in the first place.

Off-load to someone you trust

There's a reason there is a famous catchphrase of 'it's good to talk', because quite literally, it is good to talk! Keeping everything bottled up inside is the fast track to issues, and in the worst case, this can lead to depression and anxiety. Speaking about what is bothering you means you are much more likely to be able to deal with it, and if you find you allowed your emotions to burst forth, or you had a near miss, sit down and talk about what you felt and why you did what you did, with a person you can trust and confide in. Be careful who you choose, you need to feel completely secure in your confidant, and to know that they can help you with advice, or simply be a good ear to listen. Once you have done that, you will probably be able to rationalise your emotions much better.

Don't beat yourself up about it

Probably the most important point to note is that you are human, and as we have said time and time again, that means you have emotions; if you have an emotional melt-down, and afterwards you start to feel bad about it, stop right there! Yes, you had an episode of allowing your emotions to take over your reactions and behaviour, but that doesn't mean you are weak, and it doesn't mean you have failed. What matters is that you recognise it, and you do some deep thinking into the causes of the problem, and why you reacted the way you did. Everyone has a few false starts when attempting to control emotions – if it was easy then we wouldn't have to write a book about it!

It can be really distressing and upsetting to see someone you love and care about struggling with their emotions or feelings, and when you see them lashing out and having a melt-down themselves, you might feel like you are at a loss on how to help them. You can help them, but it's unlikely to be recognised at the time, so don't be upset if you don't get a thank you right away.

What you can do to help really does depend on the circumstances, and the type of melt-down they are having. Are they angry? In this case they are likely to be lashing out and shouting; it's therefore important to not take anything they say too much to heart. Are they upset? Maybe they are crying or talking a lot, and not understanding why something is happening. Again, you need to try and say the right thing here, and really be a comforting, listening ear, rather than someone who tells them what to do, and certainly not someone who judges them.

Don't take it all to heart
We've just mentioned this one, but it's really important to point it out again. Yes, words can be painful, but no, they're often not meant in the way we interpret them, and especially not when that person isn't thinking straight. Whatever comes out of their mouth, try not to react to it there and then, and if you want to iron it out at a later date, bring it up in a careful way, at a different time, preferably when they are calm.

All you will get if you say something back at this stage is abuse, and probably something worse said to you in the heat of the moment. Think about it, how many relationships and friendships are ruined because of words that were never meant? Keep this in mind and sort out any upsetting words at a later date.

Assess the situation

If you are dealing with an angry loved one, try and assess the situation, and see whether they are going to cause themselves any harm, or wind up in a worse situation because of their potential actions. If they are looking to fight, try and take them away from the scene, and if they are arguing, try and dispel the problem by subtly telling the other person in the argument to back off – in the nicest possible way, of course. It's true that they are responsible for their actions, but at the same time, if you were in that situation, you'd want your friend or loved one to help you minimise potential damage too – subtly, however.

Remember that an outburst like this is short-lived

Emotional melt-downs aren't pleasant to see, because you're watching someone you care about struggling with a feeling, allowing it to take hold for a short time. It's important to remember however, that an outburst such as this shouldn't, and won't, go on for too long.

Talk to them about it afterwards

Once they have calmed down, they're not in an emotional state, and they have recovered from everything that may have happened, sit down and have a heart to heart. You might be able to get to the bottom of what caused the melt-down, and help them deal with it, and they might be struggling to see a way to escape from their emotions, when you can. When we are in the middle of something like this, it's hard to see the wood for the trees, but another person on the outside can often see the bigger picture – consider yourself their guardian angel in this particular situation.

If you find that serious emotional melt-downs are happening on a regular basis, i.e. you feel regularly angry for no reason, or you get stressed very easily, then it's perhaps time to sit down and really assess what the root cause is. Everyone has a melt-down from time to time, but that's the key phrase to remember – time to time. If you find that your melt-downs are regular, and not just occasional, then there is a deeper problem you need to address.

Consider a melt-down to be a warning sign, an erupting volcano, but one which doesn't destroy, rather just gives you a little bit of a shake.

Chapter 7: Let's Get Practical! How to Turn Your Emotional Responses into Something Positive

If you have the mindset that you are doing something wrong if you feel negative emotions, you need to stop right now!

The fact of the matter is that you simply cannot go through life without feeling a negative emotion at some stage, and the truth is that you're probably going to feel a fair amount of negativity. What makes the difference between a happy and successful life, and one which is marred and dragged down by emotions, is how you deal with those negative feelings, and how you go about turning them into a positive.

It can be done!

Seriously, don't be so hard on yourself! You're not Superman or Superwoman, you are going to feel anger, upset, shame, or even grief at some stage in your life, probably just as much as you're going to feel joy, love, happiness, and excitement, so it's really about rolling with the punches, and changing your mindset and outlook on life.

A person who is balanced in terms of their emotions knows how to deal with negative feelings, and if you have no idea how to go about this, then this chapter will show you the way forward.

First things first however, let's look at why you will benefit from transforming those negative emotions, into positive ones.

Creativity can be found in anger

Anger as an emotion can be destructive, but it can also be very useful if you know how to harness that extreme power. We talked before about the difficulties of being able to recognise anger at the time of it happening, e.g. in the case of an emotional melt-down, but on the whole, if you feel angry, you tend to notice. If you're not in the middle of a melt-down, and instead you're simply feeling a little upset or angry about a situation, try and turn that anger into something creative. You could write about it, maybe a short story or a poem, or you could draw something, or paint. Creativity is calming, and the aim is to dispel that negative emotion, and turn it into a positive, e.g. a calm and creative feeling – you might even feel proud of what you achieved.

Difficult situations and emotions can change your outlook on life

Think about a difficult time you have been through in your life previously, did it show you a different way of thinking? Many people report that problematic and often traumatic experiences, which forced them to feel negative emotions, such as sadness or even grief, can give you a totally new outlook on life. This is a positive out of a negative, because that change of perspective could put you on a new path, one which brings new opportunities. It might sound deep and meaningful, but it's certainly a truth!

Negative emotions can help you feel empathy and compassion for others

We have talked about the fact you're going to feel negative emotions at some stage, and working through those emotions, by talking, thinking about what you're feeling, and trying to feel more positive about it, can help you become more compassionate towards other people and their upsetting situations, allowing you to feel empathy for them, and perhaps even help them. Helping others is always a positive, and will also help you feel proud, positive, and happy about yourself.

Use envy, jealousy and pessimism to spur you on to prove them wrong

If you find yourself suffering from the wrath of the green eyed monster from time to time, why not grab that monster by the horns, literally, and use it to get what you want, rather than looking at what you don't have? If you're jealous of someone because they have a better car than you, work to save up and get that car for yourself! If you are jealous of their relationship, because it seems to be happier than yours, figure out what is lacking in your own pairing, and get to work on putting things right; it's worth mentioning however that nobody's relationship is perfect, so don't fall into the trap of comparing yourself in that way!

Grief is terrible, but it can help you appreciate what you have

When we lose something or someone, the feeling is indescribable. Grief is an emotion, however over time it can be turned into a reluctant positive, by helping you appreciate what you do have. This is perhaps one of the hardest negatives to turn positive, because loss is painful, however loss is also part of life.

Acceptance is everything

Okay, so we're about to get practical and show you some ways you can help turn negatives into positives, but the most important thing to mention is that you simply have to accept that negative emotions happen – you cannot avoid them, so don't even try; what you need to do is, you guessed it, turn it on its head!

Talk it through – We mentioned this in our previous chapter about emotional melt-downs, but on the whole, talking about issues is the way forward. If you talk about your feelings, you can gain a better perspective and offload, so it doesn't all sit inside, with the potential of an explosion at a later date.

Get creative – Doing something creative, such as something craft-related, making something, drawing, painting, sewing, writing etc, will help you calm down, give you time to think things over, and it will also give you a sense of accomplishment, because you made something yourself. This is a positive.

Write it all down – Diaries and blogs are great therapy, because you can a) get everything out, and b) this gives you a record of how you feel, so you can look for patterns and triggers. We have mentioned before in this book that if you can identify your triggers or problems, you can work on the way they make you feel, and keeping a diary or blog will show you almost a flow chart of your feelings over a set period of time.

Sweat it out – We will talk about this in much more detail in a later chapter, because exercise and getting out and about is such an important part of dealing with your emotions, however for now, let's just say that dance, exercise, or yoga for instance, are all fantastic ways to distract yourself from the way you feel, and give you time to let the emotional peak pass.

Scream, scream, scream! – Head out somewhere private, somewhere in nature, and preferably somewhere that nobody is going to hear you, and let it all out. Scream as loud as you can, feel the tension and worry, hurt, and anger, whatever the emotion is, feel it coming out of your body and into the air. Afterwards you will feel relaxed, free, and probably a lot calmer as a result. A side note on this one however, don't do it in the house or anywhere public, people will actually think you're crazy!

Watch a movie that is similar to your situation – Watching someone else come through the situation that you're going through, feeling the way you're feeling, gives you a positive affirmation that you can get through it too. On top of this, watching a movie is a relaxing activity, a little bit of 'you' time, which you probably need – it's not selfish to have time to yourself, we all need it occasionally.

Make yourself feel good – Karma, whether you believe it or not, is a great way to boost your overall feeling of happiness and wellbeing, so boost your karma bank points and find a way to do something worthwhile. Perhaps you could volunteer, or donate to a charity maybe, or simply help someone who needs it. Whatever you do, if it makes you feel good, you are doing battle with negative emotions, because the positive will always win out.

Do a little soul searching – Are your emotions actually trying to communicate something to you? Maybe you're getting the answer from inside but you're not bothering to listen. Turn your thoughts inwards and have a chat with yourself – again, not literally, as people will think you are a bit crazy.

For every negative, find a positive – Turning your mind from negative to a positive is difficult, but it can be done with practice, and if you can master this, then you are on your way to hitting those negative emotions out of the park. For every single negative thought you have, find a positive and repeat it as an affirmation. Over time, your mind will re-train itself to be much more positive as a result. Don't expect a miracle overnight, but putting in the effort here will certainly lead to a brighter and happier future.

Get out into nature – There is a lot of calm to be found in the great outdoors, so find some comfortable walking shoes, grab a jacket, and head out for a walk. Breathe in that fresh air, clear you mind, grab some exercise as you go, and feel those negative emotions slip away.

Release pent up aggression – Punching someone is not a good idea, but punching a punch bag is! Head to a gym and let out your aggression in a safe and controlled way – you will feel infinitely more relaxed afterwards.

Confront the problem in a safe and polite way – Burying your head in the sand is probably not going to be the way to resolve your issues, but confronting it head on could be. Now, there needs to be some caution in place here, because if the source of your emotional problems is a person, perhaps a work colleague, confronting them in the wrong way is not going to yield the results you want; however, discussing the problem with them in a mature, adult, and sensible way could be a good route. Think about it beforehand, but facing the problem head on could be the way out of it, and therefore a huge positive.

Transport yourself to a different place – No, we're not suggesting you pack your bags and head off on holiday on a whim, although if you can, why not?! This suggestion is to find a little bit of personal escapism. Sometimes just escaping your emotions for a few hours can be the ideal way to gain perspective, so grab a book you can lose yourself in.

Friendship is everything – Make sure you have a healthy social life, which allows you well-deserved time away from your problems. Check your circle of friends are supportive, and indeed not the source of your emotional problems, and that you can trust them with anything you tell them. If you feel secure in your friendships, you really will feel supported and positive through anything.

Cultivate appreciation – Seeing opportunities rather than closed doors is a state of attitude and mind, so start trying to see the positives in life, rather than the negatives. You will find that as you move along, your emotions will begin to mirror this new mindset. In the morning, wake up and feel appreciative that you opened your eyes to another morning, and at night, look at the stars and feel happy to see them. Basically, this again may sound all very new age and deep, but having this appreciation of life and the small things, will help you become more positive, not just in your emotions, but in life overall.

Appreciate constructive criticism – If you are feeling a little defensive or hurt then you are going to feel upset by any negative comment that comes your way. The key to this is to see criticism as a building block to success, rather than someone having a dig at you. Of course, this is not an easy one to master straight away, because if someone makes a comment about your performance at work, for example, of course you're going to feel a little defensive, or even upset, but it's important to recognise this as a positive too, because you can use this criticism to improve your performance in the future, and seriously impress!

These are all ways you can turn a negative emotion into a positive, by changing the way you do things, or the way you think. You might think these are all pretty simple, but controlling your emotions isn't rocket science, it simply takes time and practice.

Try putting a few into action the next time you feel like your emotions are becoming a little too much, but bear in mind that one size does not fit all; what works for one person might not work for another, so if your friend finds walking in nature really helps him or her to declutter the mind, but you don't, there's nothing wrong with you! You might find that writing is the best therapy for you to arrange your emotions into something manageable, but another person might find it a pointless exercise. The bottom line is that you are trying, and you are doing a little trial and error exercise into finding out what works for you.

Chapter 8: How Getting Active Can Battle Your Emotions

Do you love exercise? Or do you shy away from any work out gear because you fear the perspiration that comes with it?

Well, maybe it's time you made friends with sweat and figured out the major advantages of getting active, in conjunction with managing your sometimes turbulent emotions.

The bottom line is that getting active, through sport or simply walking, isn't just great for your heart and overall wellbeing, because it has lots of cognitive and emotional benefits too. Emotional balance is perfectly possible if you throw a little exercise into your routine, and if you can find a work out buddy to help you through it, you're ticking the social life box too, and that's a major double whammy.

There are many sporting activities you can enjoy which get your heart rate pumping, such as:

- Any team sport – football, netball, volleyball etc. Playing as part of a team breeds your sense of self-worth, because working together towards a common goal will make you more confident overall, and therefore allow you to achieve emotional balance. That's an equation that certainly works!
- Yoga – An integral part of yoga, and indeed pilates, is breath, and practicing deep breathing can bring a sense of calm and balance into your life. On top of this, you're also going to be getting the major health benefits of this sporting discipline.
- Hiking/walking – You don't have to get yourself into a serious sweat to be able to grab the health and mind

benefits of exercise, because gentle walking in the great outdoors does the same kind of thing. This also has the major plus point of getting you out and about, breathing in a major lung full of fresh air too. Again, find a friend to walk with and you can chat, walk, and get some nature in your life too.

Why does exercise help with emotions?

It could be about distracting your mind for a while, allowing your emotions to abate, or it could be because pounding the pavements whilst walking, or running around and playing as part of a team, is a way to help you process what you are feeling, and label it much better than when an emotional melt-down is occurring.

Exercise, especially social exercise, is great for the mind and body, but in terms of balancing out emotions, it can give you precious time to process them, and harness their power into something useful. If you're not a sporty type in general, don't worry, you don't have to be sweating it out in Lycra, check out some of these suggestions:

- Basketball
- Netball
- Volleyball, especially the beach variety, as water is known to be calming
- Football
- Rugby
- Cricket
- Golf
- Snooker
- Darts
- Hiking

- Mountain biking
- Walking
- Paragliding
- Horse riding
- An hour at the gym, going at your own pace
- Yoga
- Pilates
- Tai Chi
- Kick boxing (fantastic for anger and aggression!)
- Swimming

None of these sporting activities are hugely high impact, and all of them will help you organise your thoughts, so you can make some sense of the way you are feeling, and gain some important clarity at the same time. This is in itself is turning your negative feelings into a huge positive, because you are boosting your heart rate, and this is always a major health advantage.

If you don't want to exercise, get social instead!

When you want to put a full stop on your emotions taking over your source of rational thinking, and you don't want to sweat it out or get sporty, you can get social instead. Now, there is a word of warning here, because drinking to excess by means of socialising can actually be harmful in terms of your emotions.

Think about your past experiences of drinking – if you were feeling angry, did you find that drinking fuelled the fire and made you feel more het up? If you were upset and crying, did that bottle of wine make you stop crying, or did it make you weep a little louder? Put simply, alcohol is a depressant, and whilst it's nice to have a drink or two with friends occasionally, or even a glass of wine to help you wind down, if you are suffering with your emotions, you may find that a drink or three takes it to the extreme, and an emotional melt-down could be on the cards.

So, if we're avoiding alcohol, or at least too much of it, but we still want to get social, what can we do?

There is the aforementioned exercise idea, because perhaps a Zumba class with friends could be a great way to de-stress, clear your head, get some exercise, and basically laugh it all out. On the other hand, there are many other social activities you can enjoy, which don't involve picking up a bottle of wine, or donning that aforementioned Lycra.

- Have a day out at the beach with friends – There is nothing more uplifting than a day out with a friend, or friends, and enjoying a day on the beach. Swim, laugh, build sandcastles if you must, but the idea is to destress from your emotions, and gain a better sense of perspective.
- Go to the cinema – Again, grab a friend and head off to see a comedy film. Laughing is a great way to feel more balanced, and it's getting you out of your own thoughts, and into the story of something else.
- Spend time with an animal – You can be social with animals too, not just people! Petting a dog or cat, or perhaps playing with a guinea pig, or watching fish, is actually relaxing, and when you're under the strain of your emotions, relaxation is very welcome.
- Join an evening class – Learning something new will give you a greater sense of worth, as well as feeling like you are achieving something. On top of this, you will meet new friends, and perhaps join a new social circle, which could open new doors for you, and eliminate the negative emotions you are feeling.

- Organise a social evening with work colleagues – If you get on well with your colleagues, socialising outside of the office is a great way to further strengthen those bonds. You could go bowling perhaps, or go and see a show.
- Organise a charity event. What better way to feel immensely better about yourself and up your karma points? Organise some sort of fundraising event, about a charity you feel passionate about, and pour your time and energy into raising funds for it. This means you will be distracted from your troubling emotions, you will boost your sense of self and self-esteem, and you will be doing something fantastic for a good cause.
- Look forward to something. Do you have a vacation on the horizon? If not, why not book one?! Having something to look forward to means you can distract yourself again, and everyone loves a vacation!

As you can see, it's mostly about distraction and giving yourself time away from what is troubling you. Emotional balance is best achieved by having a balance in your life too, and having a close knit social circle, full of people you can trust, is a great way to achieve this.

Now, let's look at a few practical scenarios of what might happen when your emotions pique, and how you can deal with it in the moment.

Chapter 9: Real Life Emotional Scenarios, And How to Deal With Them

Okay, it's all very well and good telling you what to do when you feel a certain way, but if you can't translate these tools into real life situations, then you could find yourself not really understanding that the content of this book can help you in a huge way!

This chapter is going to run through a few real life scenarios, situations where anyone would feel emotional, and situations which could pique your emotions to a higher level. We will then explore why you would feel that way, validate it, and then discuss the best course of action. Of course, we have to mention that in the heat of the moment, there could be a few off course occurrences, but on the whole, these situations will give you solid proof that the content we have discussed in this book, can really help you take control of your emotions, and therefore take back control of your life.

Scenario number 1 – The Breakup

Ah, matters of the heart; these emotions are never easy to deal with. If you have been with someone for a long time, the feeling of loss can be overwhelming, but it's important to give yourself time. Now, telling yourself that you need time is not really going to help you at that moment, but there are certain baby steps you can take, provided you can keep a sense of perspective.

The emotions you will feel – Betrayal, upset, loss, fear, worry, anxiety, desperation, anger, loss, grief, hopelessness for the future. As you can see, breaking up with someone you love can be extremely distressing.

The best course of action – It depends really on how the break up happened, whether you were to blame, whether the other person was to blame, or whether there really was no one to blame. On the whole however, the best way to deal with a break up is to disconnect yourself for a little while. You will be feeling extremely raw, and this brings up negative emotions. Seeking out support from loved ones, someone you can trust, is a great first step, because you are going to want to cry, as an emotional reaction, and you are going to want to make sense of the situation, by talking it through. We have mentioned previously that talking is a great way to achieve emotional balance, and gaining someone else's take on the situation gives you a better perspective.

Of course, time is a great healer, but telling yourself that in the moment is probably just going to make you want to roll your eyes and cry some more. Instead, take one step at a time, cry, scream at the moon if you must, but give yourself distance from the situation; who knows, the other person may come back, or you may realise that you are indeed better off without.

What not to do – Avoiding an emotional melt-down in this situation is about not contacting the other person. Your emotions will only bubble to the surface and burst forth if you get into a dialogue with the other party, and whilst you will probably desperately want to speak, to perhaps put things right, or to shout at them if it was their fault, you are only going to get yourself into a confrontation, which could mean you end up saying something you regret later.

Scenario number two – The difficult colleague

There aren't many people in life who get on with everyone they work with wonderfully well. If you find that you are popular in your workplace, and you love everyone equally, then really, you are extremely lucky. The more likely situation is that you tolerate many people, because you are paid to do so, and that you like a few others, perhaps even call them friends. If you have to deal with a difficult colleague, you may find yourself biting your tongue on a regular basis, and that can mean you start to develop feelings of resentment, anger, or even extreme dislike.

Whilst it's perfectly normal to have these emotions when dealing with someone you don't get on with, especially if they are causing you issues at work, it's important to keep a lid on any bubbling anger problems, because at the end of the day, you are paid to work.

The emotions you will feel – Anger, resentment, perhaps hate, dislike, embarrassment, annoyance, frustration, a sense of injustice, and you may even begin to feel that you don't want to go to work for that reason.

The best course of action – Controlling your emotions in this situation is imperative, because your livelihood could be on the line if you react in a negative or damaging way. The best way forward really depends on why the person affects you so much – have they actually done anything to make you feel that way? Or, is it simply that you don't click with them, and they make you feel negative around them?

In life, we have to accept that there are always going to be people we don't like, or those who we don't get along with. If you work with them, it's pretty bad luck, but unfortunately that's the way the cookie crumbles from time to time. Now, if that person has done something to upset you, and you feel like you can talk to them calmly and maturely about it, then do so; do bear in mind however, you need to pick a time when

you are feeling calm, and not when your anger is threatening
to bubble to the surface.

Calmly explain that you felt a certain way about their actions,
but that you understand you have to work together, and you'd
like to manage the situation to make it better for all parties
involved. If the situation escalates, do not become embroiled
in a shouting match, instead calmly walk away, and perhaps it
is time to discuss the problem with your manager in that case.

If however the person has actually done nothing wrong, but
you simply don't click with them, maybe you need to switch
your perspective from the negative to the positive. Try and see
the good points in the person, because there are bound to be
some, and concentrate on those, rather than the points that
annoy you.

What not to do – What you shouldn't do in this situation is
pretty obvious – do not get involved in a fight or argument.
When you allow anger to take hold, there really is never a
good outcome to be had, and the only route you are going to
go down is one of further problems, and potential disciplinary
action if you really do go too far. Stay calm, and try and
change your perspective, or tackle the problem head on, in a
calm and mature way instead.

Scenario number three – The friendship betrayal

Friends get us through some of the hardest times in our lives,
this much we know, but we also know that when we pick the
wrong friends, or perhaps when a friendship faces hard times,
there can be issues which make our emotions go into
overdrive. We pick our friends, and when they do something
wrong, we feel betrayed quite deeply. If you have a close
friend and you are betrayed by them in some way, your

emotions are likely to be quite painful to deal with. The important thing to remember here is that there are usually two sides to every story.

The emotions you will feel – Anger, hurt, betrayal, disappointment, fury, confusion, not understanding at all, disbelief.

The best course of action – Figuring out why the betrayal happened, and exactly what the betrayal is should be your focus. If you don't understand something, you're never going to get clarity or closure, and if you can actually sort out this issue, there is a chance you could save your friendship. Now, it's important to keep a lid on your emotions at the very start, because after a day or two, you may find that you feel calmer, and you're more likely to be able to sit down and have a conversation about it, rather than a screaming match, where you both blame each other for something, and end up dragging issues from the past.

Give it a few days, then approach the other person for a discussion in a neutral place. Explain your feelings calmly, and ask what caused the betrayal, perhaps even write down what you want to know, or make notes, so you get everything out into the open. If you find your emotions of anger and hurt bubbling up, take a break and breathe for a few minutes, before heading back inside to continue the conversation.

Maybe you won't be able to save the friendship, maybe it's run its course, but you should at least try.

What not to do – Pointing the finger of blame without discussing it calmly is the number one no-go in this situation. Yes, you are hurting, and yes, it's going to be difficult to keep a lid on your emotions, but that is why you should give it a day or two before you even attempt it. Space will give you time to make sense of it in your own head, to be able to see it through your own eyes, before seeking the answers you need to move forward. Also avoid dragging up any blame from the past; if you have moved on from something before, it is finished, so don't bring it up again.

Scenario number four – The loss of a loved one

This is perhaps the most difficult and upsetting situation you are going to encounter in your life, and unfortunately, 99.9% of us will experience this at some stage. Life is a constant circle of life and death, and when we lose someone who is dear to us, it can feel like the end of everything we know and love. Of course, it isn't the overall end, but it is the end of the way things are at that current time. The only thing that will really heal your emotions in this case is time, but there are certain strategies you can put into place to try and make the healing process a little smoother and easier in the meantime.

The emotions you will feel – Pain, loss, grief, upset, anger, confusion, hopelessness, a feeling of injustice.

The best course of action – Your emotions in this situation are likely to be extremely high and on edge, but the best thing to do is to accept that they are valid, and make peace with the fact that it really is okay not to be okay sometimes. There's no point beating yourself up about feeling like you're not coping so well, because everyone deals with grief in their own personal way – it really depends on how close you were to the person you lost, how they died, the circumstances surrounding it, and whether you feel like you got to say goodbye or not.

Give yourself time, and know that as the days, months, and even years go on, you will feel a little calmer and a little more able to deal with the reality. Perhaps you will never completely heal, but you will feel more able to cope as time goes on. Speaking to someone you trust and someone close to you is also a major must do, however some people feel better talking to someone who is detached from the situation, and that is why counselling could be a good route to go down if you feel that way.

What not to do – Try and avoid alcohol in this situation more than any other. Your emotions are extreme, and as we have mentioned in a previous chapter, alcohol is a depressant. If you allow yourself to become further down, you are going to find it even harder to get yourself back up. Positivity might not be something you find so easy at this time in your life, but always thinking what the person you lost would want is a good mindset to have – would they want you to be so down? Would they want you to lose control? Probably not, so honour their memory in the best possible way – by looking after yourself.

Scenario number five – When everything just seems to be going wrong

Sometimes you can't pinpoint or put your finger on what exactly is going wrong, and you simply feel like everything is getting on top of you. When this situation occurs, or rather when this state of mind occurs, you will probably feel like nothing is going right. The actual reality of the situation is that there probably are things which are going right, but that you can't see them because you have allowed your emotions to bog you down into negativity.

The emotions you will feel – Negativity, perhaps anger, frustration, unhappiness, hopelessness, upset, worry, anxiety, generally feeling very low.

The best course of action – To really come to a more positive state of mind, and to achieve true balance of your emotions, you need to pinpoint the actual problem at hand. Has something happened which has kick started this chain of negative thinking? If there has been an event such as this, look at how you can address this, and perhaps the rest of your emotions will begin to melt away. If nothing has happened, it is probably simply that you have allowed yourself to become a little down, and in that case you need to start turning negative thoughts and events into positives. Go back to our previous chapter on this, and start practicing positive affirmations, and looking for the up side of negative situations.

What not to do – Do not wade in self-pity! If there is nothing you can pinpoint which has made you feel this way, and you really don't feel like you have any issues to deal with, then it's important not to get comfortable with feeling down. Think positive, force yourself to see good things, and over time you will slowly start to feel better. It's important to mention however that if you simply don't feel better, or you notice that you are feeling worse, perhaps it's time to seek out help from a doctor, as depression is a very real problem.

These are five scenarios which most people will run into at some point in their lives, and how to deal with them. Knowing the emotions you are likely to feel will probably help you realise that nothing is wrong, and that what you feel is completely normal. Everyone feels different things according to different situations, but generally speaking, loss makes you feel a certain way, grief makes you feel a certain way, break ups make you feel a certain way – you see where we're going with this.

Look at your life currently and see if you can adopt any of these situations loosely or more firmly to what you are feeling.

If you can, adopt the 'best course of action' section, to enable you to deal with it in the best possible way. On top of this, re-read our section on how to turn a negative into a positive, and you will find that your emotions should be much easier to control and harness as a result.

Chapter 10: The End of Our Emotional Journey!

You have come to the final chapter of our little journey through that murky and sometimes confusing world known as emotions. Hopefully you will have now gained a little more perspective on why you feel a certain way about certain situations, and also why we have feelings and emotions in the first place.

We feel because we are human, and it is both a blessing and a curse to feel things so hard and so deeply. Whilst you are feeling negative emotions, it's probably going to be difficult for you to sit back and think 'wow, how lucky am I, to be alive and feeling this way', but really you are lucky, provided you can stop those negative emotions from taking control of your life, and you're able to flip them on their head and turn them into a positive.

People who are emotionally balanced don't always find this process easy, but they know how to do it, and that's what makes them live a much happier and more even-keeled life.

So, let's sum it all up.

- Emotions are normal!
- As a human being, you are pre-programmed to feel
- Everyone feels things to different degrees, and that is also normal
- There are both positive and negative emotions
- Negative emotions can lead down a murky road if you allow them to dictate your life
- Emotionally balanced people live a much more successful and happy life

- Learning to become emotionally balanced is entirely possible, in time
- Everyone feels different emotions depending on the situation, but most situations in life have a similar pattern of emotions, e.g. loss will make you feel grief, heartbreak will make you feel sad etc
- Every cloud really does have a silver lining

The ability to turn a negative into a positive is within all of us, and it's simply something you need to harness, learn, and work hard at. Your life will become infinitely better and easier if you can do this, especially for those people who really do suffer from extreme emotions.

If you are one of those people, life can become tiring, because feeling almost every emotion under the sun across the space of a day is enough to make anyone want to sleep. Whilst you might feel this is a curse, it's important to realise that you have a choice to take control, and that is exactly what this book is designed to show you.

If you want to continue your life being a slave to your emotions then you probably haven't paid much attention to the content within this book, and to be fair, nothing and no-one will make you change your mind that that case. On the other hand, if you want to be free of burdening emotions, and you want to find a way to turn those sad and sometimes upsetting emotions into something you can deal with much easier, then this book really is designed to help people like you.

By this point you should be feeling much more hopeful, and if you're not, go back and re-read it! The tools and strategies we have given you are certainly do-able, and whilst no-one is promising miracles overnight, they are achievable within a shorter timescale than you might think, provided you put your mind to it and work hard on yourself.

Having reached the end of this book you should be feeling much more hopeful, but the main points to take away from this book are quite personal. Every single person, as we have mentioned, feels things in slightly different, subtle ways, and that means that every single person who reads this book will interpret its content in a slightly different way.

Having been someone who has struggled with their emotions for many years (perhaps I blame it on the Cancerian in me), you can feel assured that the advice in this book is taken from personal experience, as well as plenty of scientific evidence.

Controlling your emotions isn't actually science, but the reasons behind why we have them is. It's important to recognise that whilst feelings and emotions can be measured to a certain degree, there are many facets of them which confuse and befuddle scientists even to this day, and their complex nature probably means that scientists will never truly understand them in their entirety. Emotions are human traits, and despite the fact that they sometimes throw up hard to deal with feelings, the fact we are feeling really does mean we are alive.

Grief is hard, heartbreak is difficult, and feeling betrayed can be like a knife has been thrust into your back, but we get through these things because we are strong, and because we are human. Nobody goes through their life without experiencing hard times, but it's how we deal with them which dictates how positive we are in the future, and the opportunities we cultivate from them.

If you only take away a few things from this book, let it be these points:

- Emotions can be hard, but they are positive because it means you are breathing!
- Every single thing in your life can be turned into a positive
- You really are stronger than you might think
- With every step towards controlling your emotions, and beating them in their attempt to control you, you will feel stronger and more able to take on the world
- Nobody in this world ever feels totally happy and totally without burden, so don't beat yourself up for not feeling like life is something from a Disney film
- If you can end every single day on a positive note, you have succeeded

I personally hope you have enjoyed this book, and that you are feeling much more buoyed up and happy having read through its content.

Remember that controlling your emotions is a journey, and it is something which is going to take time. If you feel like you need a boost in the right direction, read through the various sections of this book again, to refresh your memory. Nothing in this book is too difficult really, it's the actual practice of it which may take time and effort, depending on the severity to which you allow your emotions to take hold.

It's time to take back control of your life, holding your potential and future in your own hands, and not at the mercy of your emotions.